INTO THE ABYSS

This book is a work of accurate and true events in the life of my daughter with her and my experience with the medical and legal institutions created by our politicians. Initials are used for the names of all persons with the exception of my daughter, Maria. Everyone else I have used initials as I have for the medical facility to prevent any allegations of defamation even though none of the participants can truthfully deny anything I have written. This is so true, it's scary and I think everyone should know what happens to their family members when they don't have a power of attorney for health care in place. The powers-at-be,i.e., our so-called representatives have not legislated for an exception and all of what has occurred here is unfair and wrong to the families who have the misfortune of experiencing this abuse. Any proceeds from this book will be used for the care of Maria.

CHAPTER 1

On Dec. 19, 1962, Maria S was born with cerebral palsy. When she was 6 months old, her parents were given that diagnosis. Her condition affected her motor skills, but she excelled in school and went on to a technical college, earning a degree in accounting. She was subsequently hired by a military base in Wisconsin and worked there for several years; then against the advice of a Wisconsin government agency, applied for and received a transfer to a military base in California, where she worked for an additional 20+ years. All in all, Maria worked for the military for over 28 years. Quite an accomplishment when the experts were ready to commit her to a life of NOTHING!! Maria also suffered from depression and was hospitalized for it, but it was managed with competent medications.

1984

After graduating from the technical college, Maria secured a job with a military base in Wisconsin. She worked there for a few years, when she became severely depressed. Although she was over 21, she was hospitalized and treated for depression. Maria signed a consent form so they could talk to me. The hospital staff had no problem talking to me about her nor did they have a problem allowing me access to her. After her discharge from the hospital, Maria came to live in the same town my husband (Maria's step-father) and I lived in. We found her an apartment and she became well. While on her sick leave she went to the Wisconsin Dept of Vocational Rehabilitation asking them to help her get a job in California. The 'genius' she talked to responded with disdain; "No one is going to hire you out there. You can either go back to work at this base, or get a job here in this town at minimum wage". As I was an employee of the State of

Wisconsin, I knew what the salary of this genius was and went to him asking how would he like to work for minimum wage? Maria is not one to be discouraged or talked to like that so she got the application papers herself, filled them out sent them in and in a few weeks called me asking me if I wanted to go to California with her? I asked her for what and she said she received a call from the supervisor out there, he interviewed her over the phone, she told him she has Cerebral Palsy, the only thing he cared about was that she could do the job. She thought he offered her the job over the phone. But she told him she wanted to look at it first. I agreed to go with her so the next thing I knew we were on a plane to California. I called my husband CH, who was a truck driver and out on the road to tell him I was leaving for California. When I reserved the plane reservations, I also, reserved a rental car, not knowing I would need a credit card in my possession to take possession of the rental car. (I had never rented a car before this.) We got off the plane and went directly to the Hertz Rental desk. I tried to rent a car but with no credit card on my person that was not possible. We secured a shuttle that got us to the motel I had made reservations with. I called my husband to ask him where and how I could get some cash to rent a car. He referred me to a truck stop. Lo and behold, there are no truck stops in San Diego. I had to go to a bank. Then I called around to find where I could rent a car with just cash. I found a rent-a-wreck, called a cab to get me to the rental place, and rented a wreck. On my way back to the motel to pick up Maria, traversing the California freeway, I found this wreck had no horn and very little brakes and because there were no springs in the seat, I was practically sitting on the floor. The passenger door did not open from the outside. When I got to the motel, I saw Maria looking out the window of our room and when she saw this canary yellow wreck pull up with me driving it, she burst into raptures of laughter. Maria got into the car and we returned to the rental place where I asked for a different wreck. The attendant was very nice and gave us a much larger wreck that smelled like it had been rained on and had been drying out for several weeks in the California sun. I hoped a mouse wouldn't appear from under the seats. We were on our way to the base for her interview. Maria went in, while I waited in the wreck taking advantage of that California sun. Maria came out with a grin on her face. I asked her what happened and she said she took the job. We flew back to Wisconsin, she gave notice on her apartment, we rented a u-haul truck, my husband and I packed up her belongings, put Maria's car on a dolly in back of the truck, loaded the truck with her furniture and other stuff and drove Maria to California. Other than driving into a snow storm and running out of gas on a mountain, (my husband the professional truck driver didn't look at the gas gauge) the trip was uneventful. Maria had the foresight prior to leaving Wisconsin (not saying she didn't trust her step-dad) and filled her car up with gas, so my husband took the car off of the dolly, drove to a gas station, bought a gas can, and brought gas back to the truck and we were on our way. When we got to California we found an apartment for Maria, rented it and moved her in. She made the appointment for a driver license test, and after two tries and a few tears she passed it and had her California Drivers license. My husband and I, with tears in my eyes, flew back to Wisconsin leaving Maria in California.

CHAPTER 2

During all these years, Maria excelled in her life and in her job. She returned to Wisconsin every year for Christmas and sometimes, Easter holidays. Although Maria still suffered from depression the priest at her church and the office personnel were very helpful to Maria. In 1995, Maria was again hospitalized in San Diego. The priest called me to tell me that he and his secretary had taken her there and that she had been admitted. I flew out to see her and she was ecstatic to see me. She was worried they were going to take her someplace and I wouldn't know where she would be. I assured her that I would never let that happen, that I would always know where she is. She told me she felt safer when I was there. Maria was in the hospital for a few weeks, then was discharged and returned to work.

After a few years, Maria wanted to move out of her apartment so she found a realtor who located a beautiful Condo for her. I had invested some money for her when she was a small child so I gave her the proceeds from that investment as her down payment on this condo. I received a call from someone from the Wi Dept of Voc Rehab asking me where Maria was. I told them she had moved to California and was working for a military base. We went to visit her many times and one day while I was there she opened some mail. It was from the Wisconsin Dept of Voc Rehab telling her how happy they were to help her find the job in California. She disgustedly threw the letter in the trash. They did nothing to help her find a job out there. Upon my return to Wisconsin, I met with the director of that office and getting no satisfaction from him about their falsification of records, I met with the district director in Madison, WI. I relayed to him the incompetence of the specialist in the office of WI Dept of Voc Rehab. I gave him the complete story. With that department, as in other state agency departments, it's all about the numbers and they do anything they can to keep the numbers up for the purpose of getting as much Federal funds as they can. It doesn't make any difference how accurate their reports are. But the outrage and the truth is that Maria secured that job on her own, with no help from anyone.

After a few years in her condo, Maria decided she wanted a house, instead of a condo. She located a new subdivision that was being built, talked to the developer, contracted for a house, sold the condo realizing a $100,000 gain, put it all into the house and moved an hour away from her job. She was happy there. I helped her look and buy furniture for her new house. She was now settled and looking forward to a full life.

During the next few years, Maria became acquainted with people at her church and became involved with the organizations at the church. When a trip to Lourdes came up, Maria called and said she was going on this trip to Portugal. She went to the Shrine of our Lady of Fatima and participated in the pilgrimage to the Shrine and brought back gallons of Holy Water for all of us. Maria took a few of these trips and was participating in activities not only at her church but at work also. She made many friends and had a full and accomplished life.

In 1998 my husband and I bought a 2nd house in Arizona to get out of the cold winters Wisconsin is famous for. While in Arizona for the winter, Maria would come to Arizona every year for Easter and sometimes, if she had a long weekend, she would drive over just to spend time with us. She would also drive over to Palm Springs to see her sister, BSM and her twin nieces who were born in 2008.

CHAPTER 3

2012

Maria had worked for the military for over 28 years until June 23, 2012, when she suffered a brain injury due to a collision with a semi truck, the driver was under the influence and arrested for felony DUI. She was air lifted to a Palm Springs hospital where she was treated for a possible concussion, possible broken neck and other less severe injuries. I received a call at my home in Wisconsin from Maria. I asked her where she was and she said she was in the hospital. I asked her for what and she said she didn't know, they wouldn't tell her anything. I told her to get a nurse so I could talk to the nurse. She hollered for a nurse but no one heard her so I asked her if she could get out of bed and she said she thought so. I told her to get out of bed and go get a nurse so I could talk to someone. While she was trying to get out of bed, I heard a nurse exclaim very loudly,' oh no, you can't get up. You have to lie flat and stay in bed'. The nurse took the phone and I told her that I had told Maria to get out of bed to find a nurse. The nurse said: 'oh no Mama, that is not good. Maria has to stay in bed, we don't know if she has a broken neck or not' and then she informed me Maria had been in a motor vehicle accident and was in ICU. She had been med-flight to the trauma center in Palm Springs. I asked the nurse why they weren't telling Maria why she was there and the nurse relayed to me they had, Maria just didn't remember what they were telling her. My daughter, J and her husband K were with me when I received the call. J is an RN and also talked to the nurse finding out the technical medical information. K went on line with my computer and secured a plane ticket to Phoenix for me and car rental at Phoenix. The rest of the day and the following day I received numerous calls from Maria asking me if I had arrived there yet. I had to tell her that I hadn't left Tomah, WI yet, which is where I lived and I had to be driven to Milwaukee, WI, 5 hours south to get to the airport. I hadn't left Wisconsin yet. I told her I would be there as soon as I could and I would call her when I got to California. I arrived in Phoenix the following day. I rented the car, stayed at my home in AZ and the following day drove to California. I stopped at the State Patrol office in Blythe, California to find out about the accident. I submitted payment to them for a police report. I was given the location of her car and was able to go through it to gather up her personal belongings. I arrived at the hospital in Palm Springs several hours later and immediately went to the ICU to see Maria. Her sister BSM was there visiting her and holding her hand. Maria was in a neck brace. I gave her purse to her and when she went through it noticed that her things had been misplaced. She looked in her wallet and said that $240.00 was missing. I told her I would contact the State Patrol about it. I was able to rent a room on the hospital campus and stayed there, visiting her every day until she was released to go to her home 50 miles away. When I arrived at the hospital in Palm Springs, Maria was still in ICU and the RN informed me that Maria's friendly neighbor CM raised hell with the staff because she didn't think they were moving fast enough in performing an MRI. CM tried to get Maria to sign over power of attorney and the RN told her she had just crossed the line and to get back over it. She told CM that Maria had a mother who was arriving and she had a sister there. A power of attorney has to be signed prior to admittance to the hospital. She was on sick leave from her job at the military base. Her supervisor and office manager and other employees visited her in the hospital bringing with them a bouquet of flowers. She was happy to see them and talked about her upcoming 50th birthday which she was going to celebrate with them.

I contacted a competent attorney for Maria to do something about this accident. Maria met the attorney, and his investigator who interviewed her in the hospital, signed the contract with him and she appeared to be happy about this whole scenario. She was afraid she couldn't afford an attorney but he assured her that he doesn't get paid until he gets a settlement. She was okay with that and very cooperative.

While Maria was in the hospital, I drove to her home, retrieved her mail which was a large amount and took it to her in the hospital. The following day I went to her room to see her and her mail was gone. I asked her what happened to it and she said that she gave it to her neighbor, CM so she could pay her bills on line for Maria. I told her that was not a good idea, to give her personal information to someone other than her family. She responded that they had been friends for 8 years. The state patrol sent a claim form for Maria to fill out and sign regarding the missing $240.00. I filled it out and Maria signed it. I mailed it to the State Patrol. Maria was discharged from the hospital about three weeks after the accident. I drove her home and stayed with her for about a week setting up her follow-up appointments. We also went to the Home Depot and I bought grab bars for her bathroom, and a shower chair for her shower. We got a new garage door opener because the one she had disappeared due to the accident. We also went to a car dealership and bought a new car which was delivered to her home and put into the garage. She could not drive it off the lot because she needs hand controls to be able to drive a car. The dealer didn't do that kind of service. We also went to where the car was towed so she could see what it looked like and we attempted to get the hand controls out of the car, but we were not successful as they were not accessible. We retrieved her other personal belongings out of the car.

CHAPTER 4

After I returned to Wisconsin, Maria either called me on a daily basis or I called her and we talked about how she felt. She felt fine, she was just relaxing and her neighbor, CM, was going to color her hair for her, was helping her pay her bills on line and appearing to be a good friend to Maria. I also began keeping a daily log as to the events from the day of the accident until the present time.

The attorney, DC met with Maria at her house and explained to her the paperwork he needed her to complete for his case. She was very concerned for the truck driver that he would suffer because of her.

After I left Maria's home, I called her and talked to her. While I was on the phone with her, her friendly neighbor, CM got on the phone and said she had to talk to me about something. She said she needed to be on the phone with me and Maria so that she, CM could explain to Maria the package of papers the attorney left with Maria to fill out. I told CM that I was perfectly capable of explaining all of this to Maria myself. She responded, "How can you do that from 3000 miles away?" I told her I had done a lot of things from Wisconsin and that we were not going to continue to include outsiders in our personal business. She insisted that she should be the one to talk to Maria about all of this.

I contacted attorney DC and relayed this information to him telling him I didn't trust CM. She had inserted herself into Maria's life and appeared to be taking control. He told me that he had explained it all to Maria himself and that she understood perfectly what the papers were for and what she was supposed to do with them. He said he didn't think it sounded right, that it sounded suspicious and he would see what she was all about when he met with Maria. CM was going to drive Maria to the attorney's office for her appointment with him.

After a couple of weeks, I received a call from Maria's supervisor telling me Maria was taken to the emergency room because a neighbor found her wandering around the street at all hours of the day and night, Maria didn't know what her name was and didn't know why she had a neck brace on. I called the hospital but they refused to give me any information only to say she went home. I asked how she got home, and was told the Sheriff took her home. I called the Sheriff's office and was told only that they took her home, she refused treatment and appeared to be okay. I immediately began calling her phone and was getting no answer, and not getting a return call from Maria even though I left detailed messages. This was very unusual that Maria wouldn't return my call or call me to let me know what was going on with her. I called her friendly neighbor, CM to find out what was going on and all she would tell me is that Maria was "fine". She was irritated that the neighbor had called the paramedics. I couldn't understand her irritation because as I told her, it was obvious Maria needed help. I asked her if she had taken her medications and CM stated that Maria had forgotten to take them "for a couple of days". She was not delusional and she was "fine". I told CM to have Maria call me and she told me she didn't want to talk to me. I asked her why and she said it wasn't for her to say. I repeatedly told her to have Maria call me and her response was "what if she won't!?" Maria's brother T called Maria and CM answered Maria's cell phone. He asked to talk to Maria. CM said she didn't want to talk to him. He told CM to "put the phone up to Maria's face so she can tell me that herself". CM hung up on T.   CM had now taken control of Maria and her life. Now I am very suspicious of the friendly neighbor, CM. I'm beginning to think CM is a predator.

This began the downward spiral into an abyss of hell not only for Maria, but for the rest of her family and her friends.

I continued to call another neighbor who told me Maria was seen sitting in the other neighbor's lawn chairs all day long, in the hot sun, a lady was giving her water to keep her hydrated, Maria was standing outside at all hours of the night under a street light looking up at the sky. Her friend D went by to pick her up for church and couldn't find her she eventually saw her across the street in a neighbor's lawn chair. D said Maria had been there all day waiting for her. Maria was afraid to go into her house. D had to go into the house, wipe down all the kitchen counters, the light switches etc because Maria was told someone had contaminated everything. Also, the shower had to be wiped down and she was afraid to take a shower because something might come out of the shower. She was afraid to turn on the heat because she thought someone had done something to the gas. She wouldn't drink the water because it was contaminated and also, she didn't take her meds because someone told her not to take them because they were contaminated. Maria was hearing voices, but the information I kept receiving from her friendly neighbor, CM, was that Maria was "FINE". Maria wasn't **fine**.

CHAPTER 5

After boarding my dog I flew back out to California Mid July and met her sister BSM at a gas station and we went over to Maria's house along with a sheriff deputy but Maria wouldn't talk to us, screamed at us to "get out, why the hell did you come all the way out here?" she didn't want to see us, "get the hell out of here. I never want to see you again." I asked Maria why she didn't have the neck brace on and she said the doctor didn't think she needed it anymore. I asked her if he had taken x-rays and she said that he had not. The officers said they recognized her that they were the ones who took her home from the ER a few days ago. She still screamed at us to leave so we left and her sister BSM went back to her own home, and I rented a motel room. After two weeks in a motel room, I received a call from another neighbor, J who told me he saw Maria outside, wandering around and asked her if she needed help. She told him yes, and he asked her if she wanted him to call the paramedics and she told him she did and that she said "call my mother too". He called me and when I arrived at her house, the ambulance was there and while they were checking her out, she asked me to get her purse for her. She was on a gurney and quite lucid at this time. I retrieved her purse, gave it to her and told her I would follow the ambulance. She agreed. They transported her to the local ER. I sat in the waiting room cooling my heels for about an hour and finally asked the nurse what was going on. They allowed me into the room, and I found her crying, paging through a bible, yelling that she was not the wife of Satan and that we were all going to go to hell.

She was also seeing double. I asked the male nurse what they were going to do and he said they were sending her home. I told him "Oh no you're not"!! "She had a brain injury in a car accident and I want a CT scan." He said he would ask the doctor to order one. He returned and said the doctor wouldn't order one. I told him I didn't care what he did but she wasn't going home like this. Another nurse came over and started to ask me questions so they could write up a 51/50 which is a mechanism to get her admitted to a psychiatric facility. I went outside to call the attorney. While on the phone with attorney DC, the nurse came out and I told I him I would be there in a minute that I was talking to her atty. After I hung up with Attorney DC, I returned to the ER and the nurse said the doctor agreed to order a CT scan. While talking to me the doctor came over and asked me what kind of accident she had been in. I told him a semi truck hit her car. He visibly turned white. The results of the CT scan showed a brain bleed (subdural hematoma) and this hospital had no facilities to treat a brain bleed, so they sent her back to Palm Springs, CA where she was treated immediately after the accident. I told her I would go lock up her house and be at the hospital tonight. She said okay. She was still delusional and upset but she recognized me as her mother and seemed to be lucid at this time. The ambulance left with her and I returned to her house.

She had been in the same clothes for days, so I washed all of her laundry and gathered up clean clothes to take to her. While I was in the garage, her neighbor J stopped and asked how she was. I told him she had a brain bleed and was on her way to the hospital in Palm Springs. He told me if she needed an attorney, he had a friend who handled car accidents. I thanked him and told him she had an attorney, but he insisted I write down his attorney friend's name and phone number. I wrote down the name and phone number. After he left, I realized I would not get to Palm Springs in time to get my room on campus so I called Maria and told her that I would stay at her house, finish up the laundry and come up in the morning. She said that was okay, she was fine and would see me then.

I left in the morning for Palm Springs after calling my other children to tell them what was going on.

The hospital in Palm Springs admitted Maria into ICU and said if they couldn't drain the blood that afternoon, they would have to do brain surgery. Depending on the extent of the bleed, they would either do the surgery that night, or the following morning. I signed the papers for them to do the surgery. They were recommending this surgery because if they didn't do it, she could either have a stroke or seizures.

They allowed me to see her. I entered her room, and she asked me what I was doing there. I told her I had come to see her. She asked me why and I said I was concerned for her. She relayed that she didn't want me there and that I should go. I told her I could leave if she wanted me to and I left. The hospital called me the following day and said they were doing surgery that morning. I returned to the ICU and went into Maria's room. She asked me what I was doing there and I told her I had come to see her. The nurse said " the doctor will be in to talk to both of you." Maria stated "why does she have to be in here. I'm an adult and I don't want her to know anything about me". The nurse asked her if she didn't just talk to someone about a power of attorney, and Maria stated yes, but that she didn't sign anything. (Maria had never kept me out of her affairs before. She was always an open book to me. This attitude was not normal for her). Just then the doctor came in and asked her who her parents are. Maria responded that her parents were Barack and Michelle Obama. They took me out of the room and I asked him if I had heard correctly. He said she told them that yesterday too. I signed the papers for the surgery and left the room. Their main concern was keeping her calm so she wouldn't have a stroke.

The surgery took several hours and after the recovery, they said they got the blood out, the brain came up to where it should be and that was a good sign. Maria's sister BSM came over to the hospital to see Maria but she couldn't see anyone. While we were in the cafeteria, the surgeons came in and needed information from us. They asked us about the other scars on her head. We didn't know anything about any scars. They said there were old scars. The only scars we knew about where the ones on her legs to lengthen tendons to help her walk straight (the result of her Cerebral palsy to correct a scissors gate)

CHAPTER 6

Maria's sister BSM went up to the room to see her and Maria
screamed and hollered at her to get out. The nurses came
running and asked her who she was, she told them she was
Maria's sister. Maria was in a state of irritation and the nurses
told BSM that she had to leave, they were afraid upsetting her
would/could cause a stroke. Maria's sister left and returned to
the cafeteria where I was.

Maria was in the hospital for the next several weeks, delusional,
erratic and insisting on the O's were her parents. One day when
I called to see how Maria was, the nurse said she threw her
breakfast tray on the floor because she was angry her parents
weren't coming to get her and take her back to Wash. D.C. She
didn't want to have anything to do with me. She called me the
evil bitch. She said I had done nothing for her and that I was the
phony mother. While she was in the hospital, I stayed in the
rented room on the hospital campus. I called the nurses every
day to see how she was. She was not improving. The
psychiatrist treating her was recommending a conservator for
her because he didn't believe she could ever live alone again.
He was also trying different combinations of medication to
correct the delusions.

I called her attorney and he put us in touch with an attorney
who is an expert in conservatorships. My daughter BSM and I

signed the papers for him to act and he scheduled a conservatorship hearing with the Probate Court in Riverside County Superior Court.

One day while sitting in my rented room, I received a call from Maria asking me to take her religious medals that I was keeping for her so she could put them back on. I agreed to take them to her. I got to her room and although she wasn't very happy to see me, she allowed me into the room. I gave her the gold chain and medal. She asked where her crucifix was. I didn't know I said I would look in my purse when I got back to the room. After searching my purse, I could not find it so I called her and told her so. I told her I would buy her a new one to replace the one I lost.

She apologized to me for treating me like she had. I told her it was okay, that I understood. She was embarrassed about thinking she was a daughter of the Obama's.

While she was still in the hospital, Attorney DC came up to see her while she was using my laptop to pay her bills. He asked her if she remembered him and she said no she had never seen him before. He told her he had been to her house and she said it wasn't him, it was a different guy, his hair was different. He asked her if she remembered talking to his investigator and she said yes, but not him she had talked to three different guys.

None of that was correct. There were only two guys, and attorney DC was one of them. Maria couldn't remember these people.

The doctor called and said that he thought Maria could be discharged to go home, but I would have to stay with her for a week or so to make sure she takes her meds. I agreed to do that. I got to the hospital and Maria was happy to be going home. She wouldn't shower, saying she would do that when she got home. I had clean clothes in the trunk for her and she changed into them. The discharge process took all day and we left there about 4PM. Because Maria seemed to be recovered from everything, I called the attorney and he cancelled the conservatorship hearing. There didn't seem to be a need for a conservator anymore. I was thrilled Maria was okay. On the way home from the hospital I told her I was going to take the other highway because I was not comfortable with the freeway. Maria became upset about that and I told her I was driving and she should just stop it. We didn't get too far out of Palm Springs when Maria made a phone call asking that person to join us for dinner. When she hung up I asked her who it was, and she said CM (her friendly neighbor). Maria told CM we would pick her up at her house. We picked her up and went to an Italian restaurant. Although I told the waitress there would be two separate checks, she arrived with one check, and Maria threw out her credit card stating she as paying. I told the waitress that I would pay the check. The check with tip totaled $70. CM asked me if I wanted her money and I told her no, to forget it. Maria also asked CM if she wanted to stay over night at Maria's house and have a slumber party. I shook my head at Maria – I didn't want to sleep on the floor or the couch. CM delined. Which was a very good idea. When we got back to the house, it had been nagging on me as to why she would have a brain bleed because the doctors insisted they had ensured there was nothing going on like that when she had been discharged the first time. I asked her if she had fallen. She said yes, that CM's dog jumped on her and she fell backward, but she didn't hit her head. (I presumed this dog was a little one. I was soon to find out differently.) Just falling backward would cause jarring of the brain and could be injurious.

CHAPTER 7

While at her house that next week Maria's sister BSM and her two small children came over to visit. They drew pictures for Maria and we put them on the refrigerator. Maria was not nice or pleasant to them and when I look back on this, she appeared to be reverting to her old delusional self. I fixed a Syrian dinner and Maria was upset because I used brown rice instead of the way I used to fix it. She was upset we had only Chicken breast instead of legs and thighs. She wasn't going to eat, but changed her mind because I told her that was all we had. Barb and the twins didn't stay too long after lunch, because Maria was not pleasant to be around. They left.

That night while I was in bed, Maria came in a couple of times to make sure I was there. I told her I was, and everything was all right. The following day, Maria said her friend D was coming over, they were going to do a few things. She said D only had until 2PM. D came in and we visited in the kitchen for a while. Finally Maria said they should go because she wanted to get breakfast first. They left. Maria wasn't back yet at 4PM.

I called D and left a message asking her where they were. I got no return call. Maria finally came into the house at about 4:30PM. She came in, sat at the table with her back to me. She didn't talk to me. Then moved to the sofa and made a phone call. She asked the person on the other end if she wanted to go out to dinner that night. Oh, she said she forgot that person had other plans. Then she asked that person about going for breakfast the next day. I became pretty upset thinking that she was completely ignoring my existence so I told Maria that I thought I would go home. She smiled and said "Okay, do you want to go tonight?" Maria was very anxious for me to leave. I told her no, that I had to wait for my computer to get fixed and needed my glasses fixed first. I was waiting for new frames to come in the mail. I then told her we needed to get the mail. She got up, said she would go, she needed the exercise. After she walked out the door, I called her sister and told her what was going on. After a bit, Maria wasn't back yet so I hung up and went to look for her. She was not on the street nor was she near the mail boxes. I went to her friendly neighbor's house and asked if Maria was there. She said she was. And I asked her what she was doing there. She responded Maria needed to talk. I asked her where she was and she pointed to inside the house. She let me in and I asked her where the mail was. She said she hadn't gotten it yet, I asked her for the keys, she gave them to me and I left to get the mail. My new frames were in the mail. I returned to Maria's house. When CM answered her door, she was holding onto a large Labrador type dog. That dog had to weigh at least 150 pounds. And this is the dog that jumped on Maria knocking her down. Now it has dawned on me that whenever Maria was talking to CM, Maria's attitude toward me changed. I am now beginning to wonder if CM isn't making suggestions to Maria that is causing of some of these problems.

My phone had several messages on it from my neighbor back in Wisconsin who is an RN at the VA hospital there. I returned her call and she directed me to get out of that house tonight. I asked her what the urgency was and she said that I was a target and to get out of there tonight. I told her I was not afraid of my own daughter. She stated that she had friends who had kids like this and that they had put their mother in the hospital and that I should leave.

I packed up my stuff, packed up the groceries I had bought, called Maria's phone and left her a message that I was leaving her keys on the table and that I wouldn't be back. I left and went to a motel where I stayed that night, then went to my daughter's in Palm Springs and stayed there for a few days. The next day Maria called me saying that the voices in the house were bothering her. I told her the only thing I could do for her is go down there and get her to a hospital. She told me never mind, she would try to do this on an outpatient basis first. That's the last time I talked to her. Looking back on this, it is quite obvious the doctor in Palm Springs discharged Maria too soon from the hospital. She was not well enough to return home. And the psychiatrist she was now seeing in her home town knew nothing and did nothing for her. Although I wrote him two letters, he never responded and failed to really find out what was going on with Maria. He thought it just fine that she was happy she had no family.

CHAPTER 8

The end of August, 2012, after a few days in Palm Springs, I returned to Wisconsin. I called Attorney DC to tell him I left. After arriving in Wisconsin, I called Attorney DC to see if he had heard anything from Maria. He told me he had gotten a letter from an attorney by the name of RK to send him Maria's file. There was nothing he could do. His hands were tied. I asked him what the phone number was and when he gave it to me, I saw that it was the same number her neighbor J gave me. This is the attorney friend of her neighbor J. Now I am realizing that the neighbors involved themselves and influenced Maria in a very dangerous way. I called her neighbor J and told him that he should call his attorney friend and tell him that if Maria calls him that he should not take the case and J responded that he didn't want to get involved. I kept calling Maria but she wouldn't answer her phone and wouldn't return my calls. I called this attorney, RK and the first thing he told me was: "she's perfectly fine, the surgery fixed everything". I disagreed with him and his last response to me was that we are not doctors. I had numerous welfare checks done on her by the Sheriff's department and had called Adult Protective Services numerous times, but due to the HIPAA laws they cannot give me any feedback. The only thing the Sheriff could/would tell me is that she is "fine". After one welfare check, the deputy told me that "this is not our job. If you're so worried about her why don't you come over here and check on her yourself." I told him "because she doesn't think I'm her mother and I would probably be arrested if I were to show up on her doorstep."

Finally after his vacation, attorney RD, the expert in conservatorship matters rescheduled a hearing for conservatorship. This hearing was scheduled for November, 2012. He told me I didn't have to appear, that he would appear and let me know how it went. When I called him to find out what happened at the hearing, he said he didn't go to it.

The day after the hearing I called attorney DC and asked him what kind of an incompetent did we have here.

In December, my daughter BSM and I received a notice ordering us to appear at a hearing in January. I called attorney RD and told him about this order. He didn't say anything about it. An investigator had been appointed. This investigator refused my daily log that I had kept since Maria's accident, stating that she didn't want it "at this time". The investigator contacted my cousin F who gave her in-depth information as to Maria's relationship with me and her condition. The investigator called me and I gave her in-depth information, offering her the daily log I kept. The investigator called my daughter BSM, left her a message, but even when my daughter returned her call, she failed to respond and never did talk to BSM. She contacted my son T, and got cursory information from him. Prior to the hearing, I received a copy of this investigator's report. The report was sorely lacking and contained no information my cousin gave her, nor did it have much of the information I gave her. This report was to assist the judge in determining whether

Maria needed a conservator or not. The judge would not be able to make an informed decision regarding Maria's mental status based on this report. As a result, I filed a complaint with the investigator's supervisor, who of course, whitewashed it. My cousin also sent a letter to this supervisor along with a photo of me with Maria taken at Easter in front of Maria's house a month before this accident, which proved we were not estranged from each other.

CHAPTER 9

December, 10,2012 – my daughter-in-law AS and I arrived in California from Wisconsin. We visited with my daughter in Palm Springs, then went to Maria's house. Maria was not home. We went to the friendly neighbor's house and asked if she knew where Maria was. She responded ; "I don't keep track of her every day". AS said we were just worried about her and were wondering if she was okay. CM stated "she's fine. I've been telling everyone that, she's fine! She just doesn't want to talk to her mom!" AS said "I'm not her mom". And CM responded with: "No but SHE is!!" We left and AS commented with "what venom." CM's obvious hatred baffled me because CM didn't know me, had never held a conversation with me and knew nothing about me.

We parked up the street and waited. A car pulled into Maria's driveway and a woman got out hauling bags out of the car.

Then we saw Maria get out of the car and head toward her front door. I drove up to the car in the driveway, got out and went up to the woman. She said hello to me and introduced herself as R. (This woman is Maria's attorney's assistant). I told her I was Maria's mother. She said: "this is not a good time. She's distraught". AS asked R if she thought Maria would talk to her. R said: "let me ask her". R came back and said it was okay and AS went up to Maria. I stayed back by the car, and Maria waved me over to her. I went up to Maria and we both hugged her. I told Maria I had missed her. We went into the house with Maria. R put away the groceries. I suggested R leave so we could talk, but Maria wanted her to stay. We talked to her and R stated to me that the upcoming hearing was what was causing Maria to act like this, it was stress. I told her that stress had nothing to do with it. Maria had a brain injury, and was hearing voices. Did she know that Maria was hearing voices? She said yes, she did know she was hearing voices. R stated to me that the only thing Maria needed was to have someone to talk to and have someone to do things with. It was the stress of the upcoming hearing that was causing her anxiety. I then told her that it had nothing to do with the upcoming hearing. I was sure getting tired of repeating myself. R then suggested that Maria go to church. Maria wanted to do that and asked us if we would follow them to the church. I agreed so we got to the church and Maria was crying, praying very loudly asking God and the Blessed Virgin for forgiveness and to help her be able to pay her bills. I went out to the car and my cell phone was ringing. I answered it and it was attorney RD. He asked me where I was and told him I was in Meni. with Maria. He said he just received a call from her attorney and was told that I was knocking on the door, looking in the windows and that if I didn't get out of there he was going to call the police. I told the attorney that we were at the church with Maria and I was sick of being treated like the enemy. He told me to call the police so they have a record of it. I did not do that because I was not going to have the cops show up at the church. We were at the church for quite a while and then returned to Maria's house. I asked Maria if she wanted to go out to dinner or order a pizza. She opted for pizza. Then Maria went outside stating she wanted to visit with Robin alone. Then Maria wanted to sit out in the garage alone. While they were outside, AS said she thought she saw another set of headlights drive up. I went out the front door and saw a very tall man standing against the corner of the garage and heard the word police. I went around to face him and asked him who he was. He said "RK, who are you?" I said "I'm her mother. What are you talking about the police for?" He responded "she doesn't want you here". I stated to him: "Don't you ever threaten to call the police on me again. We will leave, but if anything happens to her tonight, I will sue **you**!" I returned to the house, got AS and we left. We parked around the corner and saw R, the assistant go past. We left and didn't get a mile away when RK called me apologizing that we had gotten off on the wrong foot and that we should return to the house. He talked to Maria and she said it was okay if we returned. We returned to the house, he left and we ordered a pizza. We ate it and visited with Maria. I asked her "why won't you talk to me?" She responded "because of what you did". "What did I do?" "You know what you did, you did it.?' AS was crying asking her what did she and TS do to her, but Maria wouldn't give an answer. During this whole time Maria showed absolutely no emotion whatsoever. AS was crying her eyes out and Maria was like an unfeeling doll. We finally gave up because she would only repeat the above statements and we didn't feel welcome there, asked her if she wanted us to leave and she said yes, so we left. We went to a motel room. The following day, we drove to Phoenix and AS got on a plane for Wisconsin.

CHAPTER 10

2013

January 8 – I received a call from Attorney RD asking me if I was going to the hearing the following day. I told him my daughter BSM and I had been ordered to appear and that yes, we were going to the hearing. He mumbled something about him not going, but maybe he would go, yes he would go to it he would see me there.

I had kept a running log of events beginning with the day of the accident until the present time. This log ran about 30 pages and I called the court to ask them how I could get this to the judge because I thought there was important information that the judge needed to see prior to the hearing. I was told that I could file it as a Declaration but it had to be done that day. The County Seat is about 45 miles from where I was staying – I made copies and took them to the court house filing them with the court.

January, 9 – Conservatorship hearing in Riverside County Superior Court, California. My daughter BSM accompanied me to the hearing. Maria was represented by a private attorney JH who knew absolutely nothing about her prior to the accident. Neither he nor her attorney RK called me, her mother, to ask what she was like prior to the accident. The hearing was held by Commissioner JB. Maria was accompanied by her 'friendly neighbor' CM. None of the testimony was taken under oath. No oaths were given. My attorney, attorney RD never showed up, instead, he appeared by phone, immediately telling the commissioner he was 'withdrawing'. She asked if there was a substitute, and he said no. My daughter, BSM and I were on our own. Maria stood with her back turned against us. She did not acknowledge us. While waiting for our case to be called, Maria and CM sat on the side of the court room, Maria's attorney sat behind them and continually conversed with CM. I found it strange he did not talk to Maria, but only to the friendly neighbor and so-called witness. When the hearing started, the commissioner berated me for submitting "ALMOST 30 PAGES" and "ALL THOSE CALLS TO THE SHERIFF'S OFFICE FOR WELFARE CHECKS????" I responded, "Yes I did. I had to know if Maria was all right. I could get no information from CM or anyone else. I also called Adult Protective Services numerous times to see if she was all right. I had to know if she was all right". I told the court I wanted conservatorship because I felt Maria needed a neurological work up due to the brain injury. The Commissioner suggested that she could order a medical evaluation but didn't know who would pay for that. I told her I would pay for it. She stated that it could run to $500, $1000 to $2000. I repeated that I would pay for that. She then suggested a public guardian and I agreed that would be okay. Maria needed help, she's hearing voices. The Commissioner responded with "'oh, a lot of people hear voices". She dismissed our concerns. The Commissioner asked CM if she had ever seen me at Maria's house. She responded, maybe once a year. She then asked CM if she had ever seen Maria's sister at her house. And CM testified "no". I responded that none of this was true. The Commissioner asked Maria if she was working and she said no, that she was on an unpaid leave of absence from work. The Commissioner asked her how she was supporting herself and she responded that she had gotten an advance on her settlement. And that she has friends and neighbors who take her to church and grocery shopping etc. The

Commissioner asked Maria if she had ever had a good relationship with "her" She responded "no". She was asked if she wanted to try and repair the relationship and Maria responded 'no'. The Commissioner then stated to me: "look at her, she won't even look at you. You can't MAKE her like you." I told her I had pictures and greeting cards from Maria to prove differently, but she didn't ask to see them. Attorney R then said, "your honor, this has gone on long enough. Her bill is getting high and......." The Commissioner then stated: "you're right, this has gone on long enough. Petition denied". The judge just put my daughter into the hands of an incompetent personal injury attorney and her neighbor who I view as a predator. CM's lies were accepted by the judge and my comments as Maria's mother meant nothing to the judge. My daughter BSM's statements meant nothing to the judge either. Maria has brain damage from an accident and how anyone can take Maria's statements as gospel is beyond me. None of these people know Maria better than me, her mother, and her sister. The Maria they see is not the Maria her family knew and loved. BSM and I left, with BSM stating to me "she's going to lose everything". That's the last time I saw my daughter, Maria. During this past year, I have been in contact with a friend of Maria's, D. She had been keeping me informed as to Maria's state of mind and Maria's activities. D is the one taking Maria to church, grocery shopping and out to eat. Shortly after this hearing D transported Maria to her doctor appointment. Maria insisted D go into the room with her. This appointment was with a psychiatrist, Dr. C. D relayed to me that he asked Maria how she was. And Maria responded she was just fine. She doesn't have to worry about PH(me) or her daughter BSM (Maria's sister) anymore. She stated she has no family and she's just fine. D also took Maria to her bank and when D was going to leave so Maria could discuss her account in private, Maria insisted on D staying with her. When the teller told her the amount that was in the account, Maria became irate and yelled that it 'was all PH's fault. She did this.' When they couldn't find the office of the doctor, Maria blamed PH. D tried to explain to her that it couldn't have been my fault because I would have nothing to do with any of that. Offices are moved all the time and how would PH know who she was going to see and how could I make them move to a different address. Maria's accusations were irrational to say the least. That same week she was seen by a Neurologist who gave Maria a letter which stated she should be getting CT scans every 3-6 months to keep an eye on her brain injury. Maria didn't think that was necessary so refused to have that done. Maria's friend D called to tell me she had taken Maria grocery shopping just before Christmas and she spent about $680. $550 of it was for gift cards for her, her friend and various other people at the church, including the choir director and the two priests. D didn't know how she was paying for all of this, but Maria was either using a credit card or debit card.

CHAPTER 11

After the commissioner denied my petition and I could no
longer help my daughter, I felt a need to write letters, so I wrote
a letter to the commissioner telling her what an injustice she
had done, my cousin F wrote a letter and sent along a photo of
Maria and me in front of Maria's house that had been taken two
months prior to the accident on Easter Sunday. I also wrote a
letter to the supervisor of the investigator with my complaining
about her incompetent and incomplete report. My cousin F also
wrote a letter to this supervisor and sent along a photo of me
and Maria that was taken at Easter just prior to the accident, in
front of Maria's house. I wrote to the chief judge with regard to
the commissioner's denial of my petition and failure to consider
my submission of photos and greeting cards Maria had given
me. With the letter to the chief judge, I sent some cards and
photos which he returned to me with a letter and three options
I had. One option was to appeal, but after consulting with an
attorney about that, found that it would be an exercise in
futility if we didn't have a doctor's declaration that Maria
needed a conservator.

Because Attorney RD didn't show up at the hearing, gave a
cursory representation of me on the phone I called Attorney DC
to ask him if he knew of anyone I could call. I told him what RD
had done and he was appalled at this. Attorney DC is no longer

in practice. He is now a judge so could not take on this accident case. He referred me to attorney MA. His former law office called MA and told him about this case. Attorney MA called me and I emailed him the information he needed regarding the accident and Maria. He was interested in this case and said I didn't need to send him any money at this time.

I have since received a copy of the police report from the California State Patrol. It is incorrect in several aspects. First the officer on the scene, although the semi truck slammed Maria's car into a call box, and he noted blood on her face and she was disoriented, asked her if she had taken any drugs. She said she had taken her medication. He then hauled her out of the car and had her perform a field sobriety test, which she failed. He sent her to a hospital for a drug test and stated in his report that she has mild MS.

Maria has cerebral palsy, not MS and she couldn't successfully pass a field sobriety test if her life depended on it due to the cerebral palsy. She walks with a cane. And his hauling her out of the car, with a brain injury could have instilled extreme damage to her. As far as I'm concerned, he used very bad judgment.

CHAPTER 12

In April, 2013 D called to tell me that Maria had called her and asked her to take her to the hospital. She thought she needed help. As D was leaving her house, Maria called her back and told her she didn't think she needed to do that. All she needed was to have someone to talk to and to do things with. This is the same thing her attorney's assistant R told me about Maria. I get the feeling that the attorney and his assistant are attempting to keep Maria from being hospitalized so they can talk her into a minimum accident settlement. A week later, April 24, 2013 Maria asked D again to take her to the hospital. D drove over to the local LL to get Maria her help. LL office staff told her they were only a day facility, but that she should go to R, CA. D took Maria to LL and when the staff began asking her questions as to her name, birth date etc. Maria was giving all the wrong information. She told them her name was Maria M Obama, her birthday was July .4. 19.... and that she was 51 years old. None of her answers added up. Maria's correct name is Maria J. S. Maria was born in December. Maria then told the doctor she didn't think she wanted to stay there and she wanted to go home. Maria told him that he couldn't keep her there. The Doctor told her she couldn't go home, that she came there for help and they were going to help her. And that yes, they could keep her. They wrote up a 51/50 which is a legal involuntary hold for mentally ill persons. Maria was admitted to the psychiatric ward of the hospital.

April 26,2013 I received a call from attorney RK, Maria's personal injury lawyer, He said that he couldn't find Maria. And in typical lawyer fashion he went on to say... "I had a doctor appointment set up for her last Friday but she didn't show up for it. I have a mediation meeting set up for this Friday and I need to communicate with her but I can't find her. She doesn't answer her phone, so I went to her house, I called the Sheriff and we got into the house, the house is fine, but Maria is not there. Her car is here so she didn't drive off somewhere. I don't know where she is and can't find her, so we put out a missing persons report". When he finally came up for air, I told him she wasn't missing. That she was in the hospital. He asked where and I told him I wouldn't tell him. I told him I had been telling them for months that she needed to be in the hospital but no one would listen to me. He responded that he needed to communicate with her because he needed her at this mediation hearing on Friday. I told him " **you can't communicate with her, she doesn't even know who the hell she is!**" He went on to tell me that as her mother I could represent her at the mediation hearing. I asked him what he was asking for and he said 5 million, but hoped to get one million. I responded that I didn't think that was going to be enough to take care of her for the rest of her life. He went on about how he had an expert financial person, blah, blah blah. I finally told him no, I was not going to do that. He was worried about the reaction of the other party because he had rescheduled it twice before. I told him I couldn't tell him what they could do with their feelings.

As it turned out, he somehow found out where Maria was because his assistant, R was visiting her. Of course, as her mother, the hospital refused to tell me whether she had any visitors or not.

Although I informed the hospital and the public guardian about this attorney, telling them they should NOT allow them any contact with Maria, as usual, the experts new best.

CHAPTER 13

I was now living in Arizona at this time, so I drove over to California and met with D who had Maria's purse and keys. I got into her house, got the mail and went through all of her papers she had on her table and counter. I sorted everything out and filed everything. Among these papers is a letter from a neurology clinic recommending Maria have a CT scan every 3-6 months. I told one of the nurses about this letter and she asked me to send it to them. I did as she requested. I called the hospital to see how Maria was. I was told she is talking to the Blessed Virgin, She is the daughter of the O's, she said she was kidnapped by me when she was 3 years old. Maria is delusional and paranoid. I informed the staff at the hospital about the accident in June, 2012. I also requested numerous times that they do a CT scan to make sure there is no brain bleed or swelling. My requests have gone unheeded. Because of their failure to look into why she is not responding to the meds, I attempted to contact the head of the psychiatry department but was not successful. I then contacted a manager at this 'world-renowned' hospital, she called the medical staff director and he was to call me. He did call me and I told him what my concerns were, he said he would meet with the doctors the next day and call me back. I have repeatedly called him leaving numerous messages and I have not heard from him. The hospital will keep her there until they can place her in a long term psychiatric facility. I called the hospital every day or so to see how she was doing. By June, it was obvious to me the meds were not working. She was still delusional, and having conversations with the Blessed Virgin. Finally, in June, I was told the nurses were instructed not to give me any information about Maria.

CHAPTER 14

While going through Maria's papers, I also found the 'advance on her settlement her attorney secured for her. These papers were signed in December, 2012. This is a loan, of $30,240.00. The $240 is a fee for the loan. The loan is depositing $3000 a month into her checking account which is how her mortgage is being paid. The interest rate on this loan is 42.4%. I submitted these papers to attorney MA for his review. I heard nothing from him about this.

I also, submitted Maria's papers for her to get social security disability. Her attorney, RK should have done this for her. Obviously he is only concerned about the personal injury and getting his cut of one third. I have talked to the Social Security office several times and gave them information with regard to her hospitalization and condition. She will never be able to work again. I also contacted all of Maria's creditors to tell them she is in the hospital and not able to pay her bills, to put them on hold until we can get control so we can pay them. The new car in her garage was 2 months behind, so I made those payments to prevent them from repossessing the car. We have too much money into that vehicle and I don't want to lose it.

He said he would get an attorney for the conservatorship and that his office advances the fees for that. I received a call from Attorney GL, who is an 'expert' in conservatorship. I told him the story about what had transpired. I also told him the hospital had initiated a conservatorship hearing for June 6. He told me to go to that hearing and ask the County Counsel to appoint me as conservator. I was to call him after the hearing.

CHAPTER 15

The social worker at the hospital told me they were looking for a court order to give Maria a drug, (Clozaril) and this is a potent drug requiring a weekly blood test to watch the white blood count.

I got to the hearing, heard someone ask the bailiff about Maria. I went up to this woman and told her I was Maria's mother. She looked at me with such disdain, I couldn't believe it. I asked her what was going on and she stated that Maria was not going to appear and that nothing would happen, that the public guardian would be given temporary conservatorship. This means they have control over her person, but not her estate, i.e., her finances. I went out into the hall to call the attorney and tell him that and ask him what I should do. I had to leave a message. I returned to the court room and found that it was all over with. There was a doctor there, Dr. P. She said 'we got what we wanted'. I asked someone what happens now. That person stated 'I shouldn't even be talking to you. Maria will stay put for now. I shouldn't even be talking to you, you have an attorney.' I left and on my way to daughter BSM, Attorney GL called and asked me what happened. I told him. He then said that they aren't going to appoint me as conservator because of some hostile relationship. I yelled at him asking him 'what the hell's wrong with those people? She's delusional. There was never a hostile relationship.'

I called Attorney GL the following day and had to leave a message. I apologized for my outburst. Actually I became unglued. I then called his friend Attorney MA but had to leave him a message. I have called several times with no success and neither one of them have called me back. I suppose my outburst was too much for them. Too bad! Stress does that to a person sometimes.

Although I questioned the public guardian's office about how Maris's bills were going to get paid, I was told, they didn't know. They couldn't do anything about her bills. They were only in charge of her person. I'm not sure what that means, because while she was under their control, they did nothing to get her treated, or get a Neurologist involved to examine and treat her.

CHAPTER 16

Maria has a new car in her garage that payments are not being made. I gave her $5000 to put on this car, along with a few thousand she had to put down on it. I did not want this car to be repossessed, so contacted the bank who is holding the loan and was told unless I am on her account, they can tell me nothing. So much privacy – all of this privacy is making me nuts. All I did was want to make the payment. I had her papers. So went on line and got the information I needed and sent them a check for two months that were behind. All of this privacy stuff is getting to me. What is the big secret anway? I even went to Maria's cell phone store to pay her bill so she would at least have a phone. The clerk I talked to told me he couldn't take my credit care unless I was on the account. I explained it all to him about Maria not being able to do anything but he insisted they wouldn't take my card. I told him he was slowly pissing me off, that he should at least make the phone call. He made the call, they took my card and I paid the bill. How easy was that?

Now I was at a loss as to what I was going to do and who I was going to get to represent me in this next hearing scheduled for July 1. I called an attorney friend to ask him about someone else and he told me to go on the internet and find one that way. I went on line and located an attorney who agreed to talk to me without a fee. Attorney A has been doing this work for 30 years and lives in the city where this hearing will be held. He knows the court, the colors of the judicial system and has a rapport with the staff. He also has a preeminent rating with a lawyer rating organization, Martindale-Hubbell. I think I found an expert. This is all good news, at least I hope it is.

I asked about the court order for the Clozoril and was told the doctor withdrew his request for a court order for this, but I was not given a reason for his withdrawal. When I was first told about this drug, I told the nurse I had looked it up on line and it sounded scary to me .She said yes, but it was known to cause miracles too. I was more hopeful after talking to her.

CHAPTER 17

Although I was calling the hospital every day and getting updates on my daughter's condition, when I called on June 20, I talked to a nurse asking how Maria was. She said she was okay. I asked her if she was still hearing voices and I was told they were instructed not to give me any information regarding Maria's condition. I would have to go through the Guardians office. They are citing HIPAA and FERPA laws. I asked her when did they receive these instructions and she said the 17th. The 17th is the day I talked to the director of the nursing staff. Now I know why he never returned my calls. I still call every day but they only tell me she's 'okay'. The hearing for permanent conservatorship is scheduled for July 1.

On June 24, I received a call from the temporary guardian in response to my call to him. I told him I had submitted retirement disability benefits papers to the hospital for the Physicians statement to be filled out and had not heard anything from them and I asked him about these papers. He knew nothing about it. I also told him I had kept a running log of events since Maria's accident and he asked me to fax him a copy. I agreed to do so. Instead I called my attorney and was told to send it to them first and they would get it to him after they reviewed it. Investigator U called me stating they had received the retirement papers now but the doctor's signature is in the wrong place and that if they get permanent conservatorship of Maria's estate, they will send the papers in. I can't think of anything more damaging than to give conservatorship of my daughter to a government agency.

CHAPTER 18

I have decided I will not cooperate with these people anymore. As Maria's mother, I should be involved in her care and treatment regardless of what she says in her delusional state of mind. If they can believe her when she says we never had a good relationship with us and they think she knows what she is talking about, why are they keeping her locked up in a psychiatric unit; why don't they ship her off to Wash. DC and the Whitehouse to live with the people she thinks are her parents? No one is giving me any information with regard to my daughter. I have cared for her for all of her 50+ years, I have been behind the scenes in making sure she is comfortable, financially secure. If one does the math, her salary was not sufficient to allow her to build a house, commute one hour one way to go to work, buy brand new cars and take trips to Lourdes, Portugal, Hawaii, etc. No one knows what her family has done for her except her family. And no one seems to want to know.

The privacy laws are a hindrance to the people who care the most for their family members. These laws were made without regard to the patients or their family members. To put one in the hands of strangers is wrong. No one at this hospital or the guardian office has asked me what Maria was like prior to the accident. They are looking at her as though she has always been like this. She was a sweet loving human being who relished her family life and relationships. Maria had a life and now because of this accident and these medical and government agencies, she has nothing.

CHAPTER 19

On June 29 I received notice from my attorney that the hearing had been continued to July 15 because one of the other attorneys is on vacation. I have made repeated phone calls to the guardian office but can get no information from them. Everyone involved with MY daughter has shut me out of MY daughter's life. On June 30 I called the hospital and asked if they received the copy of a letter from a Neurology clinic that I sent them. I was told that it would have been forwarded to the guardian office and I should call them. I called that office and had to leave a message.

On July 2, I contacted her friend D and her friend A and asked each of them if they would write up something to show that Maria and I never had a hostile relationship. Both agreed to send me something. I also contacted her friend J and left a message for her to call me back. Amazing isn't it? I am her mother and I have to prove I like/love her or she liked/loved me.

We are going to ask for a professional conservator to be appointed to care for my daughter so that I can be involved in her care and treatment.

July 2, 2013 I received a call from the guardian office asking me about my message of June 30. I told her it was about a letter from a neurology clinic and this investigator, U said they never received it from the hospital. Would I fax it to her. I faxed a copy to their office, with attention to U. This world renowned hospital is a façade. They may be world renowned for something, but I'll be damned if I know what it is. It certainly isn't in treatment of my daughter. They have done nothing for her. My repeated requests that they get a neurologist on board because of her brain injury and subsequent surgery fell on deaf ears. The psychiatrist didn't think it necessary. So much for the'expert' care. I looked up on line the doctor who is in charge of my daughter's care. His reviews are terrible and how he is still on staff is beyond me. He's also on the medical board.

CHAPTER 20

On July 5 I called the Guardian office and had to leave a message. I want to know why they and the hospital have stopped giving me information with regard to my daughter's condition. I also asked them to tell me who gave the order to the nursing staff to keep the information from me. U told me she explained all that before. I told her "no she didn't, yes I did, then explain it to me again." She said Maria won't give consent. I said "when she was in the hospital in Palm Springs, she didn't want them to tell me anything either, but that didn't matter, they kept me informed as to what was going on , I signed the papers for her brain surgery and there was no problem with any of it. What, do they have different laws for each hospital??????" U responded; "I don't know about that hospital, but we can't give any information without her consent".

A professional conservator would be to the public guardian's benefit. If they were out of the picture, they wouldn't have to deal with me because I am not going to dry up and blow away. I will be in their face every day for the rest of my life, or Maria's whichever ends first.

The laws governing mental health in this country are a travesty to the families who care and love their children, offspring, siblings, relatives. The lawmakers who have put these laws into place need to get their heads out of the sand and speak to the people directly involved with the system. Because until the medical profession insists on some sanity for the care and treatment of the mentally ill, we are all doomed. Their only concern is to warehouse these people with no attempt at treatment or care. It isn't just the mentally ill person who spirals down into an abyss of hell, it is the whole family. Maybe there were some people who abused the person, but to paint all families with the same brush and assume all families will abuse the person is not only wrong, but morally disgusting. Why should it take thousands of dollars to get the proper treatment and care for a loved one? Why should getting the proper treatment put families into the poor house. Why does the government have anything to do with personal lives? My daughter has been denied all of her rights by the appointment of a conservator. She is not allowed to even vote anymore. But she can keep them from divulging information about her to me, her mother. But in taking away her rights, they have also taken away my rights. I have a right as her mother, as her next of kin.

I have taken care of my own children for all of their lives. I have taken care of Maria for all of her 50+ years and for anyone to think otherwise or believe otherwise is themselves delusional. The medical staff want to believe Maria's statement that we never had a good relationship. If they think she is sane enough for that statement, why don't they ship her off to Washington DC and ask the Obamas to take care of her? Why don't they believe she is their child? Why do they have her involuntarily committed if she knows what she is talking about? There are too many discrepancies in this hospital's actions for me to have any trust in their treatment of my daughter. Frankly, I don't trust them.

I was so disgusted with their actions, I wrote a letter to a vice chair of the board of this hospital I never heard anything from him until several months later. He called telling me that he was going through some old mail and found my letter. How competent is his secretary I wondered. He wanted to know if she was still there, but then said that he couldn't comment as to the medical staff. He himself is a doctor. So much for this renowned hospital's full treatment of the human being. What a scam.

CHAPTER 21

July 9, 2013 I have not received a call back from my message I left for the guardian's office so I called them back. The investigator came on the phone and I asked her why, all of a sudden has the hospital refused to give me any information about my daughter's condition. Her response was that she had explained all of that to me before. I told her she hadn't and she insisted she had. I told her to tell me again then. She said it was because Maria won't give her consent. I told her that Maria has no capacity to give or deny anything. She said yes she does. That she has held long conversations with Maria. I told her if that's the case why is she still hospitalized. She said that it's two different things. Maria is 'gravely disabled' and that means she can't take care of herself. That's why she is still there. I then asked her 'so who's going to take care of her, **you?**" If they use buzz words, I guess that explains everything.

I talked to Maria's friend D and she told me she and her friend DO had gone to visit Maria on Sunday, the 7th. I told her what this investigator said about carrying on conversations with Maria and D stated, 'that's BS'. Maria doesn't carry on a conversation. She answers questions. But she doesn't converse. If you ask her a question, she will answer it. That's all. She said Maria looked like she had gained weight. That she looked healthy. Her friend DO asked her "so what else has been happening?" Maria responded that they had done a CT scan and it was normal. It looked okay and that the bruising looked like it should from the time of the accident. I will continue to ask them why they can't give me information about my daughter's condition and I will demand an answer to that question whether they like it or not.

CHAPTER 22

July 12, 2013 – I have arrived at Maria's house to prepare for the hearing on Monday, the 15th. As I was checking out the house, I found the dead bolt of the door leading to the garage to be unlocked and also the service door dead bolt in the garage to be unlocked. I had engaged both dead bolts prior to my leaving here a few weeks before. I then went around to all of the windows to make sure they were all locked and when I checked one of the bedroom windows, I saw a screen tossed against the fence. It wasn't from the window I was looking out of so I went to the next bedroom and there was glass all over the floor. I raised the shade and found the window to be broken and the screen gone. I went to the outside of the garage to look at the service door and found the metal weather stripping to be pried away from the door jamb. Someone had attempted to enter this house. I called the police and after two hours, I was still waiting for them. It's a good thing no one was in the house at the time, because I brought my pistol with me ....maybe the cops would have shown up sooner.

7/13/2013 – 12:30AM – banging on the front door. Two police officers are here. They literally scared the hell out of me. I expected them a little sooner than this, but they are here so after regaining my composure, I proceeded to tell them what I had discovered today. They followed me into the hall, and into the room with the broken window, then on to the garage to look at the damage on the service door of the garage. They took pictures and inspected the whole outside of the house. The officer told me I should get a padlock for the gate that lead into the side yard of the house. When they returned to the inside of the house they took my name, birth date, address and all other pertinent information for their records. They gave me a business card with the case number on it for the insurance company.

7/14/2013 – although today is Sunday, I called a screen repair shop and hopefully they will call back tomorrow before I have to head to the courthouse. The window will need to be repaired also. I purchased a padlock and with the help of the neighbor guy, installed it on the gate so it is not possible to be opened. One would have to crawl over the top of the fence, or bore a hole through the fence.

I have been searching for the mouse to my computer and Maria's check book. Both were on the kitchen table as of yesterday. Today they are gone. I have searched both briefcases, files, folders, her papers, desk etc and they are nowhere to be found. I was gone to church today and then to breakfast so someone could have come in here to take these things just to mess with my mind. And if that's their purpose, they are doing a bang-up job of it.

I also jammed a chair under the door knob of the service door in the garage. It will take some effort to get through that door. I also, installed an ax in the track of the patio sliding door. Hopefully, that door cannot be taken out with that in place. I'm now wondering if I should install a security camera inside the house.

I think I am losing my mind. After searching high and low for the mouse and the check book, I finally realized that I left both of those items in the house in Arizona. I have jokingly said to several people that they may have to lock me up before this fiasco is done, but I'm beginning to think maybe it isn't a joke after all. I do think I am losing it.

CHAPTER 23

I've called the hospital again to ask about Maria. The nurse was very kind and said she is about the same. She eats some of her meals in her room, stays most of the time by herself, she doesn't go to group anymore. I asked her if Maria was going to attend the hearing tomorrow and she said Maria was planning on it. Maria thinks she will win. I responded that maybe she will win me over. Poor Maria. I'm hoping she will acknowledge me and we can put an end to all of this privacy nonsense.

I am suspicious of this mental health social workers and investigator of the guardian office. They know absolutely nothing about Maria prior to her accident. All they know is what Maria herself has told them while in her delusional confused mind. I don't know how they can take any of what she says seriously. She doesn't know who she is, she doesn't know who her family is, and yet she can make decisions regarding her privacy. The only ones who are able to know anything about her condition are total strangers. None of this makes any sense to me at all.

The hearing is Monday, the 15th. This story will not end until I get back control of my own family. If there is any justice in this world, it will happen on that day. This situation didn't just mess up Maria's life, it has disrupted all of our lives. My son lives an hour and a half away from my legal residence. He has been going over every week to mow my lawn . The neighbors have been watering my flowers, my other relatives and friends have been doing what they can to support me in this.

CHAPTER 24

Well, I drove an hour to get to the so-called hearing. And justice did not happen. Maria's attorney's assistant R was there. I asked her how she came to be there. She said Maria has called her several times, she has visited Maria and gone shopping for a new outfit for her. While talking to her she told me Maria doesn't like it there, and only wants to go home to her own house. R also said she was trying to get a hold of the guardian office to ask them about bringing Maria food because she doesn't like the hospital food and she wants to ask them about getting Maria a haircut. R said she's incarcerated only without the handcuffs. I asked R what happened to the $9000 check Maria had gotten last summer for her demolished car. She said she didn't know anything about that. I told her the other attorney wrote to the insurance company because he didn't think it was enough for that car. That he had told Maria not to cash it. It was on the kitchen counter last summer when I left there. The check is now gone. The lawsuit is in limbo because Maria can't legally do anything. The hearing on Maria was supposed to be delayed so my attorney could get there. However, when the judge called the case, the public defender stated that he was tied up in bankruptcy court and had asked for a delay, but stated that he isn't a party to this case anyway, the judge agreed and went ahead with the case. Maria had not shown up so she was denied her petition to not have a conservator. There were no expert mental health witnesses. No testimony was taken and the judge then ordered the guardianship over her and also ordered the guardian to secure her house. This is not good news because I stay in her house while I am in this city for these hearings. I suppose I will be locked out of this house.

The next hearing for my petition is in August so I will be staying here until at least then.

Before heading out to the hearing, I had the locks rekeyed again and the broken locks repaired.

There is also an appointment tomorrow for the screen to be repaired and I have to get the broken window fixed. The window will be fixed tomorrow also.

I contacted the guardian office and told them that I have
secured the house. She told me I had to call back tomorrow to
talk to the deputy who was put in charge of the house. Well,
well, well, I guess I have to grovel for me to stay in a house I
helped my daughter buy. Well, whatever they do, they will not
get the keys. I had the locks rekeyed twice, to the tune of
$145.00 the first time, and $110 the 2nd time. Repairing the
screen is going to come to at least $50.00 and the window will
be $210. so if they want to reimburse me for these expenses
because they are now in control of this house, they can have
the keys, otherwise, they can rekey the locks again themselves.
I also will not give them any paperwork. If they want to know
what bills there are, they will have to do the work themselves
and find them. I am not cooperating with them in any way. All
paper is going to Wisconsin with me. When will the government
get the hell out of our lives. I don't think it will happen anytime
in my lifetime. It will just get worse. This is the biggest
nightmare that I have ever experienced. Instead of Maria
calling me or any of her immediate family, she calls
acquaintances and strangers to do for her. And these strangers
are agreeing with her to isolate her from her family. I haven't
heard yet that any of these people have suggested to Maria that
she should call her mother. I am beginning to think that in her
mind we do not exist anymore. She will have to be taken care
of by others for the rest of her life and I may never see her
again. I called the hospital and asked her nurse that if I were to
drive over there would she agree to see me and she said she
would have to ask her. I have waited for over an hour for her to
call me back. I will have to call them back I guess. I called the

hospital again and Maria's nurse transferred me to the social worker. I asked her about seeing Maria and she said she asked Maria and Maria said "not at this time". I then asked this social worker about Maria's health, I am worried she is not physically healthy. The social worker said yes, she is physically healthy. She also said that I should call the guardian office and talk to the person who has been put in charge of Maria's care. I told her about talking to R, and asking about Maria's wanting to go home to her own house. That I was going to ask R whose house she wants to go to. R isn't confined to any confidentiality laws. The social worker said that she still thinks she belongs to the O's. I guess that's the home she wants to go to. I don't think the meds she is being given are working. I don't think they care one way or the other whether she gets well or not. I think their main concern is to confiscate her assets and then to hell with Maria and her family. I question the report that the CT scan was normal. My attorney has submitted a motion for discovery to get all the documents. He's also filing a motion for the judge to reconsider her decision on his not having any standing and ordering permanent conservatorship to the public guardian. The judge did mention that on August 8th there is a successor conservatorship petition to be heard. That's for the professional conservator and me to become co-conservator. That way I can be involved in her care and treatment and the doctors will be required to talk to me. The way it stands now, they won't tell me anything about her.

CHAPTER 26

Attorney A talked to the public guardian and they will not object to our petition on the 8th. He told me he didn't think they want this case. (I'll bet they don't- not after they have to deal with me on a daily basis – even though they repeatedly tell me they can't tell me anything or give me any information about Maria, I still ask and they still give me the same answers, then I get mad and tell them what I think of their stupid laws. If I were them I wouldn't want to deal with me either.) My attorney also told me that Maria has a personal vendetta against me. I don't know what it is, but I sure wish someone would tell me. But then the confidentiality laws prevent them I suppose. Stupid laws made by stupid people, who call themselves our legislators and representatives. They certainly do not represent me. Nor do they represent the majority of the people. If the majority of the people had to live through this experience, they would throw the bums out of office, take away their lifetime pension, healthcare and any other benefits they gave themselves and throw them in prison for fraud because that's what they have done. They have perpetrated a fraud on the American people by creating agencies to take control of people instead of families being allowed to take care of their own.

CHAPTER 27

Here's another one. I just found out today because I was complaining about the lack of discipline of our children. The first thing a doctor asks a child when in his office is 'do you feel safe at home?' My kids were born in the 60's and had they asked my kids that question the answer would have been a resounding "no". Because there was so much discipline in my house they were afraid to do anything wrong, illegal or immoral. But the result was my children grew up with a strong work ethic, strong morals and a good sense of right and wrong. They did not come out of this house with the mentality that the world owes them a living or with their hand out. Nor did they become criminals. They earned their own way. Even Maria, who was born with Cerebral Palsy and had physical challenges that prevented her from navigating a college campus to such a degree that she had to withdraw from the university and enroll in a technical college where she graduated with a degree in Accounting. The campus was smaller and the students and teachers were kind. She worked for over 28 years for the military in a civilian capacity, traversing the California freeways commuting one hour each way to go to work, which required her to get up at 4AM to leave for work at 5AM, until this car accident took her life away from her and then the government tried to finish the job. Well, at least they think they have finished the job. I believe they think their power and omnipotence prevent Maria's family from being involved. One thing is for sure, God is ultimately in control and someone will answer someday for this travesty. This is no different than taking children away from their parents. The only thing is this is an ADULT child. They have labeled her as gravely disabled and as such they have taken away her rights. She does not have a right to vote, nor does she have a right to say where she lives, or who her doctors are nor does she have a right to refuse any medication they deem necessary to give her.

Chapter 28

We are all slipping further and further into the abyss of hell. The public guardian's office is now going to inventory and search Maria's house and move anything of value to **their warehouse**. I asked the public guardian if this was an indication that she will never return to her own home. Her response was that it was always a possibility of her returning to her own home. I asked her how Maria's stuff was going to get moved back to her house, would that be at my expense. She responded it would not be at my expense. I asked her if Maria knew where her home was, she responded Maria knew where it was. She also knew she was the daughter of someone else and she belonged in that city with them. Maria is quite aware of things. I don't' get it. If she is so aware, why is she still in a psych ward? Why doesn't she recognize me as her mother? Why is she trusting strangers over her own family? Why does she think she's in a state out East? Why won't they give me their diagnosis of Maria. What are they hiding? Maybe because it's something that can be fixed? But they would rather not fix it? Because her health insurance has run out, they are awaiting for Medi-cal to kick in. And because her health insurance has run out she will have to be moved to a skilled nursing facility eventually. What kind of help do you think she will get in a nursing home? None, zilch. They will make sure she gets her meds, which I'm sure are nothing but sugar pills. If they were legitimate medications, she wouldn't be the same 6 months after she walked into the place. There would be some improvement. I believe the genius doctor who is 'treating' her had given up on her and is not treating her at all. The guardian has talked to Maria about all of this and has been told of their decisions. She is in agreement with this, although she is delusional, she will believe anything any of them tell her. The guardian did say she didn't know how much of this Maria understood. They probably have told her she is going to join her family in Wash. DC.

Maria is also in contact with the personal injury attorney her neighbors found for her. She has given consent to the staff and public guardian to talk to him even though I told the public guardian my suspicions of this attorney and his 'advance on her settlement'. I advised them against allowing this attorney and his assistant to have any access to Maria, but, of course, they are in control and my wishes as her mother mean absolutely nothing. But she won't give them consent to talk to me. I am beginning to wonder what medication she is on. This attorney and her neighbor did their best to isolate Maria from her family, going to far as to ask her if she wanted them to call the police when I was there in January. His reason was that she didn't want me there. She was fine with me being there until she was alone with him or his assistant. Then all of a sudden, she didn't want me there. I am very suspicious. She is at the mercy of strangers and if this is her own doing, there is nothing I can do about it, but I can't help but think her medication is what is doing this. I believe she is being unduly influenced by others, for what reason I am unsure. I can't believe the state is after her assets. She doesn't have much and what she does have won't put a dent in their budget deficit. But I guess someone has to secure their own job and it looks like it will be at my family's expense and my daughter is the one paying the highest price.

Chapter 29

I looked up the legal code for the State of California and the Public Guardian has a right to confiscate Maria's property and funds and as they allege, 'for safe keeping'. They can also charge her estate for their 'services'. They don't, however, mention the arrest of their chief attorney who was arrested in June, 2013 for embezzlement.

Because the petition for conservatorship has been amended, the hearing is not in August, but September. I was supposed to return to WI from AZ in mid May but will now be going back in Aug. My son and neighbors have been taking care of my home in WI. This situation doesn't just affect me or my daughter, but my whole family and neighbors. I will return in Sept for the hearing and in Dec/Jan again for the winter. This legal business could go on for the next several months and my remaining here in AZ is nothing but a waste of time and money.

Chapter 30

The Guardian's office went to Maria's house on July 30 and took pictures of everything, moved everything out to put into storage. They are taking the car also. And told the person who let them in that they would be selling the house. They also brought along a locksmith and changed the locks on the house. Looks like Maria is now a ward of the state, and her family can do nothing for her or about it. Hopefully the hearing in September will change all of this. I am counting on the good Lord to help Maria and me.

Well Maria's worst nightmare has come true. Today, August 14, 2013, I called the hospital to ask how she is and was told she had been transferred out of there. No one notified me. I asked where she had been taken and they told me to a place in San B. The social worker refused to talk to me but instead told me that I had to call the Guardian's office. I did call the Guardian's office and although she apologized for me not being informed, that did little to allay my anxiety for my daughter. No one seems to take into consideration that I am her only advocate and her mother, her next of kin. I seem to have no rights in this. Although at the hearing on August 8, I understand the public defender was extremely hostile to me, even though she knows nothing about me, has never met me, nor has she talked to me on the phone. The only thing she knows is what Maria, in her delusional and confused state of mind has told her and even though Maria doesn't know who she herself is, this public defender seems to have taken what Maria has told her as gospel. Although the judge ordered the public defender to tell the social worker to call me, I have not heard from anyone. I would consider this a contempt of court citation and I will notify the judge of this lapse in following an order. It appears that the public guardian and public defender's office believe me to be an irrelevant nuisance. I raised Maria and have taken care of her for most of her 50+ years. I am not irrelevant to her or her life and situation.

Chapter 31

On August 15 I contacted the hospital to talk to Maria's nurse to see how she was today. The nurse stated; "She's been transferred out". I asked her "where did she go?" "She was taken to AH in SB". I asked "how did she get there"? "She was transported" I was devastated. Why would they not notify me where they were sending her and when? I immediately looked up the facility on line and found the phone number. I called and talked to the Director of Nursing and was told Maria had just arrived about 10 minutes before I called and they were in the process of taking her vitals. She agreed with me that I should have been notified. From the looks of the web site, the facility is an above average one and the nurse told me they would involve a neurologist, primary doctor etc. I was forever grateful that a neurologist would be consulted which is what I had been requesting all the 3-4 months she had been in the other hospital.

On August 18 I called to talk to Maria's nurse. A male came on the phone and I asked him how Maria was and he said she was okay. He then told me he couldn't tell me anything and he kept talking until I finally interrupted him and told him I needed to give him some information. I asked him about her eye and he wouldn't tell me one way or the other if it was still crossed (from the accident). I told him that it was due to the car accident and that it had not always been like that. He was very rude and demeaning to me. I guess the reports from the other hospital have me portrayed as a very disgruntled mean person. Oh well, had it been their child they would also be mean and disgruntled.

On Sunday, August 25 2013 I called A homes to ask about Maria and her nurse said she was okay and that if I wanted to talk to her there was a resident phone number he could give me. He was very nice and pleasant to me. I got the phone number and called Maria. She came to the phone and I talked to her for a while. I asked her how she was and how the food was. She said she was fine but the food was TERRIBLE. She hadn't made any friends there and I asked her if she needed anything, she said she didn't. I told her if she did to just call me and I would get whatever she needed to her. I asked her if she got the cards I sent her and she said she had. She only answered the questions I asked. There was no conversation from her at all.

In talking to the Public Guardian on August 27, she told me a Neurologist has not been included in Maria's care 'yet'. I don't know what they are waiting for? I told her the longer this goes, the more damage could be caused. She informed me that she was busy because they moved to a new office and that she was doing the best that she could. I'm afraid her best is not good enough. Her moving to a new office is a priority over a patient's life. This is a life that has been snuffed out by a semi truck driver and it doesn't look like there is a good ending to this. And the worst thing of this is that government employees are so far removed from reality that no one seems to give a rip. This is a job to them and it is no different than someone stocking shelves in a super market. It's that generic to them. None of the patients involved here are viewed as people, or human beings. They are a nuisance and a job to these employees. Shuffle the paper and move to a new office. I didn't think her first responsibility would be to move to a new office and put away her office supplies. Those are the most important things in their lives. They didn't even have the foresight to update their website with a new address and phone numbers BEFORE they moved. My letter to them was returned as undeliverable with no forwarding address. But, my daughter's mail was conveniently forwarded to their office. How conscientious of them. But packing up my daughter's personal belongings to put in their warehouse, the warehouse guys did it, and without supervision. I can't wait to see how much damage they caused. Maria had some very expensive figurines and the original boxes, which determine the value of these collectables. But, they didn't use those boxes, they used their own boxes. What happened to the original boxes for these things? Tossed out with the garbage? I'll bet. And there is no recourse, because this is a government agency and how does one sue them? The original boxes for collectables determines the value of these items. She may need all the dollars she can get for these things to pay for her care. As broke as California is, I don't understand their lack of concern to readily put her on the government tab. Nothing has been said to me as to what they did with her pension papers. I guess that's not a priority either. They would rather have her living off of the taxpayers. The incompetence of this agency is unbelievable.

In Mid September, 2013, after I had submitted an email with my concerns to the administration of this Public Guardian's office, I received a call from a manager, deputy director or director, I'm not sure what her position was, but she was calling me with regard to my concerns. I immediately asked her about the boxes for Maria's figurines. She said she talked to the Warehouse staff and they didn't see any boxes. I told her I had taken pictures of everything in that house and had a picture of them. She requested I send her a copy, which I did. Then I told her about Maria's pension and potential health insurance from her employer had they submitted the papers like they were supposed to. She was going to check into all of that. Her real concern about the boxes was that someone else had access to Maria's house. (I sent Maria's friend from church the key so she could let the Public Guardian into the house for the purpose of 'securing' it against loss or damage.) I doubt Maria's friend stole the empty boxes. What a stupid suggestion!! During my conversation with this manager or whatever she was I did tell her that I had worked for a government agency for 20 years and that I know how people are hired, the caliber of people that are hired and how they work, and frankly I don't trust many of them. And if I don't hear a favorable response from this person, I guess my suspicion extends to her also.

I received a call from this administrator telling me she had a photo of the figurines in a Styrofoam box and it sounded to me like it is an original box. She offered to send me a picture of it and I told her it was all right, I would get it later.

The conservatorship hearing is now set for October 7, 2013. That date is in my religion, 'The Feast of the Most Holy Rosary'. As a Catholic, we put a lot of faith and trust in the power of the Blessed Virgin Mary. I left Wisconsin on Monday morning Sept. 30 and arrived in Arizona on October 2. On the 3rd, I went to Urgent Care and was diagnosed with bronchitis. I had to be in Calif for the hearing on the 7th so the doctor loaded me up with strong meds to get rid of this infection.

I arrived at the attorney's office at 11AM on October 7 and was told we are not going to the hearing. The professional conservator and his attorney will appear and we were told not to go to it for fear of screwing up anything. That I should call his office about 3-4PM to find out what happened.

AT 4PM I called Atty A's office and was told the professional conservator was appointed and that I should call him to find out when to meet him and where.

I called Mr. LD's office and talked to him. I am to meet him tomorrow at 11AM at the atty A's office.

October 8, 2013 I arrived at 11AM to meet with LD, the professional conservator. I provided him with all the pertinent documents he would need for Maria's care. He told me the psychologist and doctor testified that Maria is no different than she was a year ago. Obviously she has not been treated. He will get a psychologist and neurologist on board to get her the treatment she needs and he is going to try his hardest to get her back into her own house with a caregiver within 6 months. I sure hope he is successful with this. He will also retain a personal injury attorney who knows what he is doing. The attorney her neighbors found for her is incompetent, inept and unethical and we will get rid of him as soon as possible.

It's a sham to have the public guardian's office in charge of anyone. They failed to get her any treatment and were only concerned with paying her bills with her own money and moving her personal effects out of her house and into THEIR warehouse. They refused to reimburse me for the repairs I made to the house from the illegal break in. And they refused to include me in Maria's treatment and care or inform me as to Maria's medical condition. What good they are is beyond me and ditto for the medical people charged with her so-called 'care'. There was no 'care'. They take an oath to 'do no harm'. Where is the oath to 'do responsible care'.? I even called Maria's insurance company to report the medical charges as fraudulent. Her insurance company was charged $215.00/day by her so-called physician. I was told that if he reads the chart, he can charge. Wonderful, he doesn't really have to DO anything. He just continued to charge every day until her insurance ran out, then ship her off to a nursing home under the expense of the California taxpayer. I think this deserves some investigative reporting from CBS, NBC, or ABC. Where is Chris Mathews? Where is Chris from Dateline? I think instead of reporting on sexual crimes, I think they should report on crimes against humans being such as these. Because what I have described above is certainly a crime.

As this past year was unfolding, I wasn't sure whether or not Maria and the rest of my family would ever climb out of this abyss of hell. However, with a professional conservator on board, I am sure we are all going to be all right. I thank God for the Judge who ruled on this and could see the truth. Only time will tell and I hope I live long enough to see it. My fear that Maria would die in a place with no family around because government employees knew what was best for her over her own family will not be realized. My fear that I will die before ever seeing Maria again or knowing that she is acknowledging me as her mother will not be realized either. With someone who cares and is compassionate taking charge of Maria, I know she and the rest of my family are going to be okay. The government thought they knew what was best for Maria, but they certainly didn't know what was best for Maria, me or my family.

Now that a professional conservator is in charge and the public guardian office is not, they still manage to screw up the works. They are now demanding that the professional conservator remove all of Maria's personal belongings from their warehouse within 10 days and they will not release her finances to him until he has accomplished that. I interpret that as blackmail. Blackmail is a crime isn't it? They also returned her October social security check to the Social Security Administration. I can't help but wonder where they find these people to work in such an important and responsible position. It must take personnel/human resources quite an effort to hire people who know nothing. The hearing was on Oct. 7, her social security check arrived prior to the hearing. Why the hell didn't they deposit that check into her checking account or give it to the Professional Conservator once it was ordered that he was now in charge? Why send it back????? It's not that she's not entitled to it. And now how does her mortgage get paid and the car???? This is incompetence at its worst or rather stupidity on the part of the lawmakers who drafted the law. I received a call from the Public Guardian's office concerning my complaint to them about the above snafu and was told once they were taken off of the guardianship, the law required them to reverse the social security payment and as a result, it is returned to the social security administration. Also, IF the professional conservator needs funds to remove Maria's furniture and other things from their warehouse, they will release her funds to him. My response to that was of course he's going to need funds to move her stuff. They can't expect him to use his own money for that. Talk about mismanagement of funds. That is exactly what this is. How long will it be before she gets her check?

I worked all of my life in one capacity or another and had I worked at my job like these people work at theirs, I wouldn't have lasted a week. It isn't the legislature that has to be replaced but I would say most of the government employees usually called bureaucrats. We are in dire need of a change all the way around.

www.ingramcontent.com/pod-product-compliance
Lightning Source LLC
Chambersburg PA
CBHW070606290526
45790CB00002B/799